Dr. King's
Simple Guide to Holistic Health:
Lessons Learned
From My Personal Journey

Dr. Elizabeth King

ISBN: 0615639569
ISBN-13:9780615639567

Library of Congress Control Number: 2012939032
DRK Global Enterprises, INC., Fort Lauderdale, FL

Dedication

To my beautiful daughter, my miracle child, Elizabeth, my why for living.

To my mother and hero, Andrea, who taught me how to be a survivor and live life to its fullest.

To my three sisters and best friends, Sandra, Miguelina and Altagracia, who have been my role models and who in the hospital never allowed anyone to see me without my lipstick.

To my "Mama," who until her dying day took care of me.

To my entire family and all of my friends, who have always been there for me.

And last but not least, to my wonderful and patient husband, John, who has stuck by me through being bed-ridden, opening up a holistic center, and writing this book.

Table of Contents

Preface
by Dr. Gladys T. McGarey

The United States of America is known worldwide as the leader in health care. We spend more money on it than any other country, so why do so many people feel the system is broken and needs to be fixed?

There is no question that we have the best emergency- and acute care-delivery system. We know how to take care of diseases, but in the process, have we forgotten the individuals who have been diagnosed with the diseases?

Two people may be diagnosed with the same disease, but the way each manifests that diagnosis is unique. So why do we think we have to treat it the same way, when we know a medication may cure the disease for one person but could be toxic for another?

Pharmacies are required by law to print up all the adverse reactions a drug can have because people react differently. Yet these therapies are still being used to treat people with a variety of diagnoses.

There is little recognition that curing a disease is not the same as healing a person.

We need a paradigm shift in what we think healing really is and how we can go about having it happen. Here are three nursery rhymes that help us understand this problem.

One:

There was an old woman
Who lived in a shoe
She had so many children
She didn't know what to do.
She gave them some broth
Without any bread
And whipped them all soundly
And put them to bed.

Conventional medicine is like the old woman. She is tired. She is old, and new things—children—are hard for her to deal with.

She lives in one shoe, which is like our health care system. You can't go anywhere in one shoe. The whole system is stuck and can't move.

She had so many children: The children are the multitude of diseases and the therapies that are supposed to heal them.

She didn't know what to do: The diseases and therapies are out of control. The system doesn't know what to do.

She gave them some broth without any bread: The system tries to control the diseases by giving them therapies that are inadequate. They work for the babies—acute illnesses—but do not have enough of the bread of life to work for chronic long-term diseases. The system is stuck with the diseases and has not even considered the people who have them.

And whipped them all soundly and put them to bed: All she knows to do is to quiet the symptoms by punishing them and putting them to sleep. It is like attacking pain and then giving pain medicine, so it doesn't bother us.

Two:

Mary had a little lamb
Whose fleece was white as snow
And everywhere that Mary went
The lamb was sure to go.
It followed her to school one day
Which was against the rule.

It made the children laugh and play
To see a lamb at school.

Here is where holistic medicine steps into the picture. We are now dealing with a real person. She even has a name, Mary, and that name has power.

Mary had a little lamb: She had divine, living energy that was hers alone.

The lamb's fleece was white as snow: It was pure, alive, young, and healthy.

And everywhere that Mary went the lamb was sure to go: She could not get away from this energy. It was always with her. It belonged to her. No one could take it away from her, and no one was in charge of it. She was in charge of her own healing. This is significant. A surgeon can repair a wound, but the person does his or her own healing.

It followed her to school one day: This healing energy even follows us into the school of life.

Which was against the rule: The business lives we live have rules that discourage us from bringing this living energy into the workplace. But Mary and her lamb are clever, and they manage to get into school anyway. When that happens, it makes the children laugh and play.

To see a lamb at school: These children do not act like the children (diseases and therapies) in the old woman's shoe. They are engaged with life and living, so they don't need to be punished and put to sleep. When the symptoms of our diseases are looked at for the messages they bring, and when we are engaged in our healing, we can learn from the symptoms. Healing can happen so that the person is healed and the disease may, or may not, be cured.

Health and wholeness are possible even when disease is present.

Three:

Humpty Dumpty sat on a wall
Humpty Dumpty had a great fall
All the King's horses
And all the King's men
Couldn't put Humpty
Together again.

Humpty Dumpty sat on a wall: Humpty Dumpty represents our current health care system. It has been sitting on a wall encased in its own shell, not at all engaged with the life of real people. It has felt secure and above the rest of the world. Isn't this the way conventional medicine has seen itself for many, many years?

Humpty Dumpty had a great fall: Our health care system has fallen and is broken. Perhaps it fell because a great wind came and blew it down. People are beginning to take back their power and have caused a great change. Change can be a great wind.

All the King's horses: For many decades, our presidents have been trying to fix this broken system.

And all the King's men/couldn't put Humpty together again: Even Congress has been trying to repair this broken shell. They can't, of course, because the shell is dead. It has no life of its own. Our health care system has become so broken, it cannot sustain itself.

But there is hope! Inside that egg is a living chick growing and waiting for the right time to hatch. Humpty Dumpty had to fall off the wall so the shell could be broken open and release the new life.

Real life manifests on the ground, where its roots can deepen—not up in the air. This chick or new life is named Living Medicine or, as some prefer to call it, Holistic Medicine. Whatever its name, it is strong and healthy. It just needs to be protected and nourished.

What Dr. Elizabeth King has done in this wonderful book is to provide the tools and wisdom necessary for us to awaken to who we can be. We must no longer content ourselves with being stuck in an old shoe.

It is time for the Mary in each of us to get back into the school of life with our little lambs and age into health. The tools Dr. King gives us in this book will help us achieve a life of health and wholeness.

Gladys T. McGarey, MD

Dr. McGarey is widely recognized as the "Mother of Holistic Medicine." She is internationally known for her pioneering work in holistic medicine, natural birthing, and the physician-patient partnership. Her work through her foundation, The Gladys Taylor McGarey Medical Foundation, has helped expand the knowledge about and application of holistic principles through scientific research and education, and the foundation is helping to bridge the gap between traditional and holistic medicine. Currently, Dr. McGarey and her foundation are actively involved in health care reform.

INTRODUCTION

I wrote this book because I know what it feels like to be in excruciating pain, to be sick, or just to want to be healthy but not know where to start. I, for one, did not have a clue about how to begin my journey back to health (read my story on page 1 to see how I got there). Everything I did I had to struggle to learn on my own, which is not easy when you don't feel well. I vowed that after going through my journey—from living with chronic pain to living a drug-free, joyful, and healthy life—I would share my story and knowledge so that no one else would have to experience what I went through.

This is a primer on holistic medicine. It is written for the skeptic as well as the believer. It is meant to be a good starting place to begin your journey of taking back your health and your life. If you have questions along the way, email me at DrKing@

DrElizabethKing.com or go to my website at www.
DrElizabethKing.com and read the "Frequently Asked
Questions" section. I also would love it if you shared
your success stories by emailing them to me.

WHAT YOU SEE
MAY NOT BE WHAT YOU GET

Everywhere you look these days, you see the terms
"holistic" and "wellness"—in TV ads, on billboards,
and in books and magazine articles. Well, you can't
believe everything you read.

People with no credentials whatsoever are throwing
these terms around because the concepts are so popular. Everyone desires to be well, and who doesn't
want to be holistic? Isn't that the opposite of scattered
and broken?

That's all good, of course, but you need to look care-
fully and see the difference between people who use
"holistic" and "wellness" as meaningless come-ons,
and people who are dedicated to using them correctly
to benefit the rest of us.

A lot of misinformation about holistic medicine has
been put out there. In this book, I am going to point
out the misconceptions and replace them with facts.
First, I want to address ten of the myths I hear almost

daily from patients who come in believing they are true.

Here goes:

MYTH: Holistic medicine is the same thing as alternative therapy. Under this definition, "going holistic" means turning away from any conventional medical options and using alternative treatments exclusively.

FACT: Although "holistic" and "alternative" are often used interchangeably, holistic medicine includes both conventional and alternative medicine. Holistic is closer to the term "integrative" than it is to the term "alternative."

MYTH: Traditional or conventional medicine is the best approach to treat whatever ails you.

FACT: Often, conventional, or allopathic, medical doctors treat the body and ignore the mind. Typically, traditional or conventional mental health professionals treat the mind and ignore the body. Conventional treatments typically do not address the spiritual. Often, conventional medicine treats symptoms with drugs or surgery rather than looking for what causes the symptoms. Humans are mind, body, and spirit. Therefore, the best approach is to use holistic medicine, which addresses the mind, the body, and the spirit.

MYTH: Holistic medicine is airy-fairy—not accepted by conventional medical doctors.

FACT: Many different types of health practitioners, including medical doctors, embrace holistic medicine. For example, hypnotherapy has been used by dentists, as well as doctors, for more than a century. Many of the treatment options under the umbrella of holistic medicine are well researched by reputable institutions. Just make sure you do your homework.

MYTH: Holistic medicine refers only to alternative healing practices.

FACT: Holistic medicine is the fusion of all treatment options, both conventional and nonconventional. Its quest is to find the underlying causes of symptoms, rather than just covering up the symptoms with drugs.

MYTH: Holistic medicine addresses only the mind and spirit.

FACT: Holistic medicine addresses the whole person: mind, body, and spirit. These three components are viewed as intertwined. Drugs and surgery are promoted only as last resorts.

MYTH: Holistic medicine is witchcraft.

FACT: Once you understand that holistic medicine is the fusion of conventional and nonconventional treatment options, you know that it is not witchcraft.

MYTH: "Spiritual" as used in holistic medicine means "religious."

FACT: Spiritual refers to the essence of the person you are—your core. Holistic medicine views spiritual betterment as vital to healing.

MYTH: In holistic medicine, the practitioners are in charge of your medical care and they do all the work.

FACT: In holistic medicine, you and all of the practitioners on your team are partners. You are encouraged to educate yourself and engage in self-care.

MYTH: Holistic practitioners do not believe in ever using medicine or surgery as a treatment protocol.

FACT: A true holistic practitioner looks to incorporate all treatment options, including medicine and surgery, if that is what the patient needs. Drugs and surgery are usually not the first treatment options. Nutrition is usually the first option.

MYTH: Holistic medicine includes only treatment options such as homeopathy, acupuncture, hypnotherapy, meditation, vitamin supplements, exercise, oxygen therapy, Reiki, herbs, aromatherapy, yoga, nutritional counseling, colonics, biofeedback and organic living.

FACT: Holistic medicine does incorporate all of the above, but it also includes medicine, surgery, epidurals, and other types of conventional and nonconventional medical and wellness care.

A disclaimer: Please be aware that not everyone who advertises the practice of holistic or wellness medicine is reputable, licensed or trained. When you search for a holistic practitioner, you need to be proactive and do the legwork, check your own state's licensing or certification requirements, go to professional associations for references and ask for personal references. It's just like getting references for a good doctor. Although you can be pretty sure MDs have the right credentials and licenses, having them doesn't necessarily make the MDs reputable.

Later in this book you will find a glossary of holistic terms. The contents are for educational and informational purposes. They should be used only as a starting point to seek out a professional who is qualified to conduct the selected treatment. The United States runs on health care. Especially given the aging Baby Boom population, medical topics are a great preoccupation for the vast majority of Americans. If you yourself are not the focus of concern, you're worried about your kids, your parents, or your community.

How could it be otherwise? Health care costs are astronomical and growing. In this general election year, Medicare is constantly in the news.

These statistics from the U.S. Centers for Disease Control and Prevention tell the story:

- Heart disease, the number one cause of death in 2009, claimed 599,413 lives that year.

- Cancer was the primary diagnosis in 28.2 million visits to physicians' offices and hospital outpatient and emergency departments in 2007.

- Patients with major depressive disorders spent an average of 6.8 days in hospitals in 2009.

- For the years 2005–2008, 48 percent of Americans had used at least one prescription drug in the past month, according to a 2010 report.

Chronic pain is a whole other source of staggering statistics. The American Academy of Pain Medicine reports that in 2011, at least 116 million U.S. adults had chronic pain conditions, a number that doesn't include children or episodes of acute pain. The painful cost to society is at least $560–$635 billion a year, or, about $2,000 for each U.S. resident. And in 2008, federal and state governments spent \$99 billion on medical procedures for pain.

So if you suffer from chronic pain or a serious disease or condition, you are not alone. You may be where I was five years ago, when I was misinformed and skeptical about holistic health. Like most people in mainstream America, I believed that there was only one route to health and that this generally involved medication and surgery.

I thought "holistic" meant nonscientific, airy-fairy stuff. When anyone dared to recommend an alternative or nonconventional treatment for my chronic pain, I would conjure up images of hippies chanting in a circle. Don't get me wrong—I love hippies (my older sisters were hippie wannabes in the 1960s), and I've always been jealous of their ability to walk barefoot on hard pavement. But I certainly didn't believe that chanting would get rid of my pain.

Now, I will be the first to admit I was naïve, and after reading my story, you will understand why I say that. I believe that what happened to me was not a coincidence. I needed to survive a dark time in my life so I could help others understand that the body is well equipped with all the tools to self-heal; it just needs some assistance. A holistic approach to health and wellness will provide that assistance.

Don't feel ashamed or embarrassed that you accepted all the negative propaganda about holistic medicine. Just admit it and move on with an open mind. Since you are reading this book, you must be someone who is ready to learn—or at least you're curious enough to browse.

My Story

•

I had survived polio and thirty-five operations, but I was pretty sure I couldn't survive this.

For two years, the pain had been getting worse and worse. It was a struggle to walk with crutches. I can't begin to tell you how desperate I felt to be confined to a bed because of the excruciating pain throughout my body. I thought I would never walk again.

It was hard to believe my life had come to this. Not long before, I had been a vibrant, productive, highly motivated and successful person.

My orthopedic surgeon, Dr. David Padden, a Johns Hopkins–trained physician, was my champion.

This was the same doctor who had done my total hip revision in 2000, when, because of the complexity of the surgery, no other doctor would touch me.

He went through hell and back with me, trying to figure out the puzzle of what was going on and why I wasn't able to get better. Constantly encouraging me to not give up, he tried everything within the scope of his practice and referred me to the best available specialists.

He shared my disappointment when nothing worked. Pretty much all I got from all those other specialists was another prescription for pain medication and the prognosis that I would never get better. After seeing more than ten doctors who couldn't find the root of the problem, I was convinced that I had cancer but no one was finding it. Seriously, it felt as if a large tumor in my back was trying to break through my skin right underneath my left shoulder blade.

By the time Dr. Padden sent me to see yet another back surgeon, Dr. John Coats, I was actually praying that he would be the one to find the cancer so at least I would know what was wrong with me. But when Dr. Coats walked into the examining room where I lay, fearing more bad news, to give me the results of all the scans he had ordered, he said something totally unexpected: "You don't have a tumor, and I don't recommend any other surgery. Your problem is that all of the surgeries you have undergone have finally taken a huge toll on your body, and now your muscles are all contracting. You need to think about alternative medicine, like acupuncture."

I did not have an epiphany right away. "Alternative medicine" meant nothing to me; I was a skeptic about acupuncture and anything else that sounded New Age-y. I said nothing, but looked at Dr. Coats as if he had a horn sticking out of his head.

Finally, he broke the long silence with a question that changed the course of my life forever: "What do you have to lose?"

All my life, I've beaten the odds. The youngest child of a single mother of five, I contracted polio when I was 3 years old. By 1963, vaccines against the disease were available in the United States, but they were not available in my native country, the Dominican Republic. I was one of thousands of children who were part of the polio epidemic. Most of the children died, and the ones who survived wound up in iron lungs for the rest of their lives. Or, if they were lucky like me, they just ended up with their limbs atrophied and paralyzed.

My mother, a courageous, independent, and progressive young woman, had just gone to the United States in search of a better life for her family when I got sick. "Mama," as we affectionately called my grandmother, stayed behind to take care of the five of us, and her other two children, while my mother went to get everything ready in the States for all of us to go live with her.

In the beginning, my doctors didn't know what was wrong with me. First, I was quarantined in a hospital room with a lot of other very sick children. Then, I was given to my grandmother so that she could take me home to die. The doctors told her there was nothing they could do.

With just a glass window between us, I remember seeing and hearing, as clear as if it was yesterday, my grandmother crying and the doctor saying, "She is going to die."

Thank God Mama never gave up on me.

My grandmother had to break the bad news to my mother over the phone. I can't even imagine how hard that must have been–to tell my mother her little girl was dying. To add to my mother's desperation was the fact that she couldn't come back right away because she was waiting to be granted permanent status.

4

If she came back before she had her green card, it would ruin our chances of ever coming to the United States.

She waited patiently for her immigration status to allow her to come back to get us, which probably took more than six months. Her goal was to get me to the United States as soon as possible for better medical care. Meanwhile, all she could do was work three jobs to send money back home to make sure we were all taken care of. She wanted especially to make sure my grandmother could get me the best doctors.

After a long, hard road of intensive physical therapy, I recovered most of the use of my body. The polio had impacted my entire left leg and my right foot. I wound up wearing a big metal brace that went from my hip to my feet, and big heavy boots. I had to learn how to walk again, one step at a time.

In 1965, my mother was finally able to bring us to live in New York. Fast forward three years, when I was 8 years old and had the first of what would be more than thirty operations on my legs.

Thanks to my powerhouse of a mother and my grandmother, I never really knew I had a disability; it was more like an inconvenience. My mother would make me do the same chores my sisters had to do. If we were painting, and I was wearing my leg cast, she would sit me on the floor, hand me a brush, and say, "Your job is to paint the baseboards."

Miss O'Connor, my special education teacher for grades two through five, was another powerhouse in my life. She also instilled in me self-confidence and gave me the ability to see past my disability. I guess that is why I have never let my "inconvenience" prevent me from doing anything I wanted to do. I just knew I needed to work harder and smarter to accomplish my goals.

My older sisters have always been there for me. Throughout my life, they have been my best friends and my protectors. After every one of my operations, when I was old enough to wear makeup, they were the ones who made sure that as I was being wheeled out of surgery, I had my signature red lipstick on. They knew how important that was for me, because it was the symbol that I was alive and well.

I spent most of my growing-up years in a body cast in a hospital. By age 14, I was walking fairly well and my big, heavy brace was replaced by a smaller, plastic one that came to just below my knee. At 17, I had my hip fused and was told I would have a difficult time walking. That was the last time I spent almost an entire year in a body cast.

Somehow, I managed to get back on my feet again. The next year, I graduated from high school with my class. Freed from the cast and hungry for independence, I moved to South Florida all by myself at 18. I married four years later and had my daughter when I was 23.

My daughter was, to me, a miracle child. With my small frame and medical history, I had been told I probably would never have children. When Elizabeth—yes, her name is also Elizabeth—was conceived, I was ecstatic. Three months into my pregnancy, I almost lost her. I was put on bed rest for three months, but I didn't care as long as she was OK.

Then came this most perfect human being in the whole world, this little person who changed my life and gave me a reason to live.

Over three decades, I earned a bachelor's degree in education, a master's in social work and a doctorate in education leadership. I pushed myself up the ranks to administrator in the Broward County, Florida, public school system, one of the nation's biggest.

In 1996, while working as a middle school counselor in Pembroke Pines, Florida, I underwent a total hip replacement. Four years later, I had to have a total hip revision on the same hip because it had collapsed under the heavy weight of the prosthesis. After a lot of bone grafting, my muscles were weakening, and I was in constant pain. At times when I sat, my hip would dislocate; my gait slowed, and my limp got more severe.

The recovery time was brutal. I was completely dependent on my husband, even to go to the bathroom. He would sit on the floor and push my feet one step at a time, while I struggled with a walker.

It took me almost two years to return to work full time, but I did it. I never really recovered fully, and I needed to take pain medication frequently to function.

In 2005, I fell getting off an elevator and tore my meniscus, the disc that cushions the knee. Relatively simple surgery would fix it, but for me that thirty-fifth operation marked my return to a pain-filled life. It was deeply depressing to realize I had become a victim, a label I had fought my whole life to avoid.

I hit a wall just as I was reaching the height of my career as an educator and mental health professional, overseeing about twenty-five dropout-prevention programs for the Broward County school board and running workshops at the state and local levels. I was accomplishing on a grand scale what I had always felt was my mission: advocating for poor children and families.

Now I couldn't get past the pain that kept me from achieving anything on behalf of children. I was taking eight to ten pills a day just to survive, and I spent most of the time in bed sleeping.

My family suffered, too. Elizabeth was away at law school, but my stepdaughter was living with us. She was impacted because her dad was dedicated to taking care of me. My sisters and my mother were flying back and forth, trying to give my husband a break. Everyone was concerned about my emotional and physical state. I was effectively bedridden and unable to work at the school board. Little did I know that I would never go back.

After two of the worst years of my life, I had reached the point that when Dr. Coats asked what I had to lose, I had to admit the answer was nothing.

Dr. Coats conferred with Dr. Padden, who agreed I should see an acupuncturist. I put my life trustingly in his hands—and God's—and made the call.

It was the start of my journey back to a productive and happy life.

After just one acupuncture session, I felt relief from the throbbing pain I had suffered for almost two full years. I cannot express how elated I was. There was hope for me after all!

Soon I added massage therapy and started reading about other alternative treatments for pain, including hypnotherapy. By then, I was cutting back on pain medication, but I still had to take a couple of pills per day to function. Combined with these treatments, the spirituality that gave me hope during the tougher times was now helping me regain my health.

I resolved to do whatever I could to get rid of the pain once and for all. I was already drawn to hyp-notherapy because I was a licensed psychotherapist and was curious about the mysteries of the mind. So I traveled with my husband and daughter to Santa Cruz, Calif., where I trained as a hypnotherapist.

After completing the certification course, I re-turned to Florida and added self-hypnosis to my rou-tine of acupuncture and massage therapy. I used self-hypnosis to bypass the pain signals.

I had always thought I ate well, but I started to really educate myself on nutrition and what causes in-flammation. I came to understand the correlation be-tween diet and how I felt physically and emotionally. I changed my diet and immediately started to feel the difference in my pain level. Also, the swelling in my feet went down significantly.

In less than four months, I was able to eliminate all pain medication. I returned to being a fighter and a lover of life. I still occasionally experience pain— you don't endure thirty-five operations without feeling residual effects—but when I do, I just return to the recipe that got me back on my feet again. Of course, since then I have added quite a few other staples to my regimen of pain relief, like the Ondamed® and taking my Juice Plus+® (you will read about those two treatment options in the glossary portion of this book).

I am living proof that a holistic approach to health really works. I still do not take any pain medication.

To this day, I continue seeing Dr. Padden because I trust his guidance. He led the team that took a comprehensive, holistic approach to my health. I shall always be grateful to him and the other doctors who were willing to get out of their comfort zone and encourage me to seek treatments that are typically considered nonconventional.

As I look back, my only regret through all of this is that I wish my mother and I had known about all of these treatment options before. It may have saved me from having a few of the thirty-five surgeries, and for sure it would have saved me from much of the pain.

All I had to endure to finally get the help I needed led me to open a holistic center, write books, give lectures, host a radio talk show, and speak to anyone who could benefit from holistic healing. It is my way of paying it forward.

I believe it is my calling to use my talents as a teacher and mental health professional to bring awareness and offer hope. Whether you choose acupuncture or hypnotherapy or any other treatment is beside the point. I just want you to realize it is all here for you.

If, after reading my story, you're still skeptical, think of what Dr. Coats asked me: "What do you have to lose?"

HOW TO USE THIS BOOK

This book is meant to be more than a guide for you to begin your journey toward holistic health. It is also meant to be used as a workbook. After teaching for almost twenty years, I know the importance of being able to take notes and highlight. To make it easy, I have provided you with blank pages at the end of this book so you can take notes and jot down websites, personal goals, or questions as you read along. Go ahead and chicken scratch and highlight to your heart's content. I give you permission, so give yourself permission. If you have questions, you may email me at DrKing@DrElizabethKing.com. I can respond to general questions, but I am not allowed by law to give out specific advice. Still, I will respond and guide you.

This book is filled with information, ideas, techniques and resources. It is meant to be used, so use it! Get out there and start your journey by putting together a great team of holistic practitioners who will take care of you as a whole person.

If you do, it will change your life. I promise.

Abundant blessings,

Dr. Elizabeth King

GLOSSARY
OF HOLISTIC TERMS

Here are the building blocks for a holistic approach to health and well-being. As with any building, the trick is putting the blocks together solidly and correctly. Each collection of blocks must be chosen for you individually—some will help you, others will not. It's up to you and your team of holistic practitioners to sort through all the options and to focus on the best plan for you. This is just a partial list of holistic assessments and treatments; there are hundreds, if not thousands, more. The goal of this book is to get you started on the path to understanding that there is so much more to improving health than just medication or surgery. It is up to you to take it upon yourself to continue learning about the different options you have for prevention and healing.

Acupuncture

Procedures that use needles or electricity to stimulate anatomical points. Practiced in Asian countries for thousands of years, acupuncture is based on the premise that the body is a blend of two opposing forces, Yin (the passive principle) and Yang (the active principle), and that when they fall out of balance, pain and disease result. The imbalance leads to blockage in the flow of vital energy (qi or chi, pronounced "chee") along a network called meridians. The flow can be restored by using acupuncture at points on the body that relate to the thousands of points on the meridian matrix. Acupuncture is commonly used to treat conditions of the bones and muscles, and many kinds and sources of chronic and episodic pain—lower back, neck, headaches, joint, dental, and post-operative. Many practitioners use it as a treatment for other conditions, including post-operative nausea, allergies, fatigue, depression and anxiety, digestive disorders, infertility and menstrual disorders, and insomnia.

Allopathic medicine

The conventional or mainstream system in which medical doctors and other health care providers respond to symptoms and diseases with standard treatments such as drugs or surgery. "Allopathic" comes from the Greek words "allos," meaning other or opposite, and "pathos," meaning suffering or disease. Allopathic medicine is a disease-management system that focuses on attacking the body part that shows signs of acute illness.

Aromatherapy

The use of essential oils for healing. Essential oils are taken from the roots, leaves, seeds, and blossoms of plants and used in concentrated extracts. The mix of ingredients determines what each essential oil is used for, and the oils are inhaled, massaged into the skin, or poured into bath water. Some are treatments for physical conditions, while others promote emotional wellness through relaxation or pleasant smells. Essential oils have been used therapeutically for almost six thousand years. The modern science of aromatherapy dates to 1928, when French chemist René-Maurice Gattefossé discovered that a burn he suffered in a lab explosion could be healed with lavender oil. Aromatherapy has been used to relieve stress, anxiety and depression. Essential oils used by qualified midwives have helped women in childbirth. Other conditions aromatherapy may help relieve include indigestion, premenstrual syndrome, hair loss, constipation, insomnia, the pain of rheumatoid arthritis, the itching side effect of dialysis, and psoriasis. Basically, there is an essential oil for every condition.

The important thing to note is that not all essentials are created equal. To receive the most benefit, make sure the oil is classified as "therapeutic medical–grade oil." The cheaper oils are usually combined with pre–servatives and additives. Try to stay away from that type of oils because they may cause skin irritation.

Biofeedback

A relaxation technique in which you learn to use your mind to control bodily functions such as heart rate and blood pressure. Electrical sensors connected to your body help you receive and measure information, or feedback, about your body. You monitor small metabolic changes such as temperature, heart rate and muscle tension. The sensors teach you how to make subtle changes in your body, like relaxing certain muscles, to achieve results such as reducing pain. Biofeedback can be used to help treat anxiety and stress, asthma, the side effects of chemotherapy, constipation, high blood pressure, incontinence, irritable bowel syndrome, pain, and a multitude of other conditions.

Chiropractic

A method of bringing the spinal cord into alignment after it has been misaligned as a result of physical trauma, poor posture or stress. Chiropractic practitioners use a variety of techniques, but mainly they perform adjustments to the spine or other body parts. The goals are to correct alignment problems, get rid of pain, and improve function, relying in part on the body's self-healing ability. Many people turn to chiropractors when they experience back pain, particularly involving the lower back.

Colonics

Also called colon cleansing or colonic irrigation, the use of an internal bath to wash away toxic waste lining the walls, pockets and kinks of the colon. A professional administers the bath using pressurized water and hydrotherapy equipment. The bath is like an enema in concentrated form, and each one is the equivalent of four to six enemas. The treatment is used both to prevent disease, and for illnesses and conditions such as constipation, psoriasis, acne, allergies, headaches and colds.

Counseling

An intervention used by a trained psychotherapist, psychologist, or other mental health professional to help solve life's problems, giving the patient a sense of happiness and control. This usually involves increasing self-esteem, improving relationships, avoiding or limiting uncomfortable experiences, and developing effective coping skills to deal with trauma and negative thoughts and behavior. Psychotherapy can be short-term, with just a couple of sessions, or it can involve many sessions over several years. Sessions can be one-on-one, or with couples, families or groups. Through psychotherapy sessions, you may learn what caused your problems so you can take control and solve them; learn how to identify and change negative thinking and behavior; explore relationships and experiences, and develop ways to improve your decision-making; learn to set realistic goals for your life; and learn how to cope with physical and psychological pain.

Craniosacral therapy

A form of noninvasive and drugless chiropractic manipulation used by osteopaths, massage therapists, naturopaths and chiropractors. Also called CST and cranial sacral bodywork, the treatment was developed in the 1970s and 1980s by osteopath John Upledger based on a discovery by William Sunderland at the turn of the 19th century. The idea is to stimulate the body's natural healing process by gently using the hands to evaluate and kick-start the craniosacral system. This system is comprised of the membranes and cerebrospinal fluid that surround and protect the brain and spinal cord. Craniosacral therapists have reported success in treating stress; neck, back and chronic pain; migraines; the side effects of chemotherapy and radiation, and other medical problems associated with mental and bodily dysfunction.

EMDR

An abbreviation for Eye Movement, Desensitization and Reprocessing; protocols used to reduce the negative effects of traumatic memory. Research shows they are an effective treatment for post-traumatic stress disorder (PTSD). The treatment stems from an observation made in 1987 by psychologist Dr. Francine Shapiro: Under certain conditions, eye movements can reduce the intensity of disturbing thoughts. During traumatic events, the combined efforts of the left and right sides of the brain to process and neutralize information are stymied, resulting in "frozen" memory. The traumatized individual may experience repetitive symptoms commonly associated with PTSD, depression, panic attacks, insomnia or anxiety. EMDR helps neurologically, as well as emotionally, to "unfreeze" the memory and promote wellness.

Health Fusion™

A protocol developed by Dr. Elizabeth King. It takes integrative medicine to another level by not only combining different treatment options but actually fusing them. A perfect example would be using hypnosis and acupuncture on a patient at the same time. The benefits of both treatments are enhanced. The choice of which treatment options will be fused depends on the patient's needs. As of this writing, formal research has not been conducted to confirm the effectiveness of this approach, but results achieved at the International Holistic Center speak for themselves.

Homeopathy

The use of natural substances—taken from plants, minerals, or animals—to promote wellness and cure disease. It is based on the idea that "like cures like," the principle that the body can heal itself when the sufferer is given very small doses of a highly diluted substance that produces similar symptoms in healthy people. Homeopathy was conceived by the physician Hippocrates in Ancient Greece and developed more than two-hundred years ago by a German physician. The term comes from the Greek words "homeo," meaning similar, and "pathos," meaning suffering or disease. The treatment is highly individualized, and is based on physical, emotional and mental symptoms, as well as genetic and personal health history and body type. Common remedies include red onion, mountain herb, and stinging nettle plant.

Hypnotherapy

Techniques enabling the practitioner to bypass the conscious mind and reach the subconscious. The mind enters a state much like deep meditation, and the patient can restructure thought processes, change behavior and build willpower. In this state, the patient can find greater clarity as to needs and desires, look closely at unresolved personal experiences, and become more open to change. Hypnotherapy is used to quit smoking and other addictions; lose weight; control blood pressure; and reduce or eliminate pain, stress, anxiety and depression. It is also used to overcome phobias (fear of flying, of public speaking, etc.), help heal skin diseases such as warts and psoriasis, improve self-esteem, and enhance athletic and business performance. Change can happen only if the patient wants it to happen. The patient does not lose self-control unless that is the patient's desire.

Integrative medicine

The idea of treating the whole person—not just a disease—through conventional Western medicine, along with nonconventional or complementary techniques. Integrative medicine took on a higher profile in the United States after a major 1993 study showed that one in three Americans had used an alternative therapy at some point. Integrative medicine, geared to promoting health and preventing illness, is one of the touchstones of the holistic approach to body, mind and spirit.

Life Coaching

A singular relationship between a board-certified Life Coach and a client that is geared toward identifying the client's goals and developing a plan to achieve them. The Life Coach is not a mental health professional licensed by the state, and the process should not be confused with counseling. The coaching relationship, based on mutual respect and trust, is a confidential partnership that enables the client to make informed decisions about work, relationships, home life, and the future. Close to half (42.6 percent) of participants in the 2010 International Coach Federation Global Consumer Awareness Study, all of whom had experienced coaching, said their motivation was to "optimize individual and/or team performance." In a 2009 survey of coaching clients, 96 percent said they would work with a life coach again.

Live blood analysis

The instant analysis of a few drops of capillary blood taken from a fingertip and viewed under a powerful microscope that is connected to a camera. The process is also called live blood cell analysis, nutritional microscopy, or darkfield microscopy biological terrain assessment. Unlike a conventional blood test, the analysis is in real time, giving the patient the opportunity to see his or her blood on a video screen and to participate in the examination of his or her body. The condition of red blood cells may be an early warning sign of stress and disease that may eventually manifest itself. The objective of live blood analysis is not to diagnose disease or to sell nutritional supplements, but to find imbalances in the blood's pH levels that may require further investigation. In the short term, the patient works with a qualified nutritional microscopist to identify any nutritional needs or excess acidity and toxins, and to formulate a healthy eating plan to address these challenges.

Lymphatic drainage

A type of massage that enhances circulation in the lymphatic system by helping to drain it. The lymphatic system is a network of vessels, tissues and organs that aids the body in regulating fluid balance and fighting infection. It takes excess fluid, called lymph, from the tissues and returns it to the bloodstream. Lymph drainage therapy (LDT) practitioners use their hands in wavelike motions to assess the lymph flow and thereby determine the best routes for draining stagnant fluids, and then gently encourage that movement. The result is improved overall circulation. Therapists have reported success in detoxifying the body; relieving inflammations, chronic pain and the symptoms of chronic fatigue syndrome and fibromyalgia; aiding relaxation, and improving vitality and memory.

Magnetic field therapy

The use of magnets to help diagnose and treat physical and psychological disorders, relying on the connection between electromagnetic energy and the body. Practitioners believe that the earth and other electromagnetic fields interact with and change the body, and that for optimal health, the body's electromagnetic field must be balanced. Magnets, which are always applied to the outside of the body, are either electrically charged to deliver a pulse to the treated area, combined with acupuncture needles to treat energy paths within the body, or left on the treated area for some period of time. Magnet therapy is used to treat joint problems like arthritis, migraine headaches, episodic and chronic pain and depression. The Ondamed® is one example of an electromagnetic frequency machine.

Massage

Manipulating the body's soft tissue by hand or with a mechanical device. All types—including Swedish, Deep Tissue, Therapeutic, and Raindrop—involve kneading, rubbing, brushing, and tapping the muscles and connective tissue. The goals are to improve circulation and detoxify, to reduce stress, and to enhance wellness. In addition to aiding circulation and relaxation, massage can ease tension headaches and migraines, carpal tunnel syndrome, sciatica, tendonitis, arthritis, fibromyalgia, post-surgery adhesions and swelling, depression and anxiety, immune dysfunction, chronic pain, pregnancy and birthing, sports injuries, neuralgia and cancer-related symptoms. It can also help get rid of scar tissue and stretch marks.

Meditation

The union of body and spirit by self-directing attention to focus on the mind's inner sanctum. Meditation is an ancient mind-body process that employs concentration to make the body relax and the mind become clear and calm. The various techniques for achieving this include mantras, imagery, and breathing control, and the practitioner may be passive or actively engaged in movements such as walking or the Japanese martial art of Aikido. Regular meditation can enhance both psychological and physical wellness by relieving stress, and has been used to treat anxiety, high blood pressure and cholesterol, chronic pain and substance abuse. It may also help maintain a high quality of life for people who have cancer.

Nutritional counseling

One of the most underrated aids to health in conventional medicine. In the United States, medical doctors and mental health professionals seldom ask what the patient is eating. If you think about food as the fuel of the human body, it makes total sense that nutrition should be discussed at the doctor's office.

Nutritional counseling is vital to lifelong wellness and for treating physical and psychological problems. The first step to wellness should be testing for food sensitivities that can result in illness. The body can react badly to manmade chemicals such as food dyes and sulfites, and to naturally occurring chemicals like solanine, tyramine and MSG. After testing, a diet can be tailored to individual needs, perhaps by adding herbs and food supplements. Some supplements are macro-nutrients (carbohydrates, fiber, fats and proteins), and some are micro-nutrients (vitamins, minerals and trace elements that are manufactured rather than naturally occurring). Nutritionists may also recommend whole-food-based products such as Juice

Plus+®, with its natural nutrients from seventeen fruits, vegetables and grains in concentrated form.

The nutritional counselor may be a registered dietician, a doctor of Oriental medicine, a medical doctor or a certified nutritionist. In addition to losing weight and keeping it off, nutritional counseling may help the client with conditions like chronic pain, fibromyalgia or migraines; may help the client increase energy and mental clarity levels, and may help the client improve his or her appearance and look younger.

Ondamed®

A device that uses frequencies and weak-pulsed electromagnetic fields to create a therapeutic response in
the patient's autonomic nervous system. Non-invasive
and painless, it is based on the principle that humans
are electromagnetic beings who are receptive to electromagnetic vibrations. Ondamed is a Latin term meaning "wave medicine," and Europeans started using it
twenty years ago. The technology locates dysfunctions
by scanning the body for disruptive frequencies. Then
it provides the stimulus to return the body to the correct
frequency and heal itself. Using the process of pulse
biofeedback to identify each body's optimal electromagnetic frequencies, Ondamed jump-starts natural
cellular repair and regeneration by inducing subtle current impulses in fluids, organs and tissues. The temporary stimulation, prolonged by the patient's partici-
pation, promotes relaxation, muscle re-education and
rehabilitation to achieve a state of complete wellness.
Ondamed's pulsing fields break through the blood-
brain barrier, so they improve the absorption of phar-
maceuticals, nutrition, hormones, etc.

Organic living

Living simply, healthfully and close to nature; avoiding drugs, hormones and synthetic chemicals. This philosophy encompasses everything from food to clothing to home and work environments. Organic farming produces food naturally, without synthetic chemical fertilizers, harmful chemical pesticides or genetically altered organisms to boost crop yields. The idea is to make zero impact on the environment, to protect limited resources, and to produce safe and healthy food. Organic ranchers and dairymen do not use drugs or animal hormones for their livestock. Supporters of the organic lifestyle say food produced this way tastes better and has higher nutritional value. Primitive man used organic methods before the discovery of chemicals. These compounds saved time and improved crop quality, but had disastrous effects on our air, water and soil. The recent return to organic farming occurred when consumers started rejecting toxins and pushing for higher health and environmental standards.

Oxygen therapy

Changing the body's chemistry for the better by providing it with extra oxygen. Normally, your lungs absorb oxygen from the air, but some conditions, like chronic obstructive pulmonary disease, can keep you from getting enough oxygen. Injured tissue needs even more oxygen. In hyperbaric oxygen therapy, the patient breathes pure oxygen in a pressurized room. As the blood carries oxygen throughout the body, it stimulates the release of growth factors and stem cells, which promote healing and fight infection. A well-established remedy for scuba diving's decompression sickness, oxygen therapy can also treat serious infections, persistent wounds from diabetes or radiation injury, carbon monoxide poisoning, crushing injuries, gangrene, burns, skin or bone infections that cause tissue death, and severe anemia.

Dr. Elizabeth King

Pain management (holistic)

Using holistic treatments to alleviate acute or chronic pain. Doing so means combining conventional options, such as medicine and surgery, with nonconventional options, such as acupuncture, hypnotherapy, herbal medicine, biofeedback and the Ondamed®. The goal should always be to start with the least invasive and drugless approach, because side effects accompany medication and surgery. Another important aspect of holistic pain management is nutritional counseling, which can help pinpoint a patient's dietary choices and patterns that cause inflammation. Nonconventional therapies facilitate recovery, prevent additional health complications, and improve an individual's quality of life. Chronic pain and acute pain from an injury, illness or surgery, respond well to nonconventional pain-management treatment options. The key is to find the right practitioners and the right combination of therapies.

Don't be discouraged if your program doesn't work right away. Holistic pain management is about healing your body, and that takes time. Unfortunately, Americans have been conditioned to expect immediate results because they usually respond to pain by taking a pill. The drug may eliminate the symptom, but it doesn't resolve the underlying problem. Besides, every person is unique and a person's pain should be treated uniquely. You can always try more treatment options and specialists, so don't give hope. It's just a matter of putting together a great team that works for you.

It is important to pay close attention to the psycho-emotional aspect of pain, as it is debilitating both physically and emotionally. The patient may feel depressed, anxious or hopeless. These intense emotions may contribute to the patient experiencing more pain. It is vital that the patient speak with a mental health professional to process his or her feelings and build coping skills.

ReflexologyAn ancient Chinese technique that uses pressure-point massage to increase the flow of energy throughout the body and restore balance. Reflexology is based on the premise that since reflexes in our hands, feet and ears connect through the nervous system to every other body part, stimulating the hands, feet and ears increases circulation and improves blood supply, and may alleviate stress and other health problems. Adapting an early form of the method, called "zone therapy," Eunice Ingham developed reflexology in the 1930s. The technique has been used as a preventative, to cure sleeping disorders and sports injuries, and to improve mental alertness, creativity and productivity, as well as to enhance the relationships among body systems.

Reiki

A centuries-old Japanese technique to reduce stress and promote relaxation and healing. The term combines two Japanese words—"rei," meaning "God's wisdom or the higher power," and "ki," meaning "life force energy." In Reiki, the practitioner uses the palms of the hand to transfer healing energy to organs or glands, or to help balance bodily chakras, also called energy centers. Feelings of peace, security and well-being are said to flow from the treatment, which can be a tool of massage therapists, chiropractors, nurses and all others who employ touch to heal. Reiki is offered at about 15 percent of U.S. hospitals, including the Memorial Sloan-Kettering Cancer Center in New York and the Dana-Farber Cancer Institute in Boston, according to Consumer Reports on Health.

Spirituality

One's inner connection to a higher power. The source may be religious, or not. It may come through meditation or another medium. Whatever the channel, spirituality creates a sense of wholeness and a transcendent affiliation with universal life forces. The spirit is what sets each individual apart, like DNA but without molecules. It must be nurtured, and the way in which this is done varies from person to person. For some, music feeds the spirit; for others, it is reading or anything that expands the mind. An artistic expression may be spiritually based. The goal of holistic health is to integrate the mind, the body and the spirit. The impetus to overcome illness is often associated with an individual's inner strength, and the wellspring for that strength is spirituality. Since the dawn of time, people have been searching for answers to the mysteries of life and death, and have turned to religion and other forms of spirituality to find them. Dr. Elizabeth King's professional experience and research confirm that healing correlates with having strong spiritual beliefs.

Thermography, or Digital Infrared Thermal Imaging

A safe, noninvasive, radiation-free diagnostic technique that uses an infrared digital camera to track surface temperature and vascular changes in the body. The result is an early warning system for cancer and other serious diseases. The technology also reveals preexisting conditions like arthritis or diabetes, and identifies the chemical and inflammatory activities that could signal acute health problems such as strokes. Each body has a unique internal roadmap, much like a fingerprint. In breast or full-body thermography, an ultra-sensitive, infrared digital camera captures these images and produces a detailed, color-coded map of the body. The first images serve as a baseline; subsequent scans are taken. Then the images are analyzed and compared to reveal abnormalities. It is recommended that other scans, such as a mammogram or MRI, be done along with thermography. Breast thermography technology has been FDA -approved since 1982.

Vibrational and sound healing

A hands-on, heart-centered therapy that opens gateways to the soul and heals at the cellular level, harmonizing the body, the mind and the spirit. The multidimensional clearing process helps heal patterns that are blocking you from wholeness, happiness and success. The practitioner talks with the patient to uncover core issues. Next, the two participate in an empowering, energy-releasing session that transforms unwanted patterns and the residue of past experiences. Most patients say they emerge with feelings of forgiveness, compassion, lightness, joy, relief, greater insight and a general sense of well-being. Vibrational and sound healing helps reduce stress and anxiety, and supports and promotes self-empowerment, better relationships, mental and emotional clarity, self-love and creative energy. The treatment has received scholarly attention as part of the ongoing research into Parkinson's disease.

Yoga

Application of ancient Indian Vedic teachings to exercises that—combined with controlled breathing, relaxation, meditation, and diet—unite a person's physical, mental and spiritual elements. The word comes from the Sanskrit root "yuj," which means, to join. Physical exercises are called asanas, or postures. Yoga therapy is an emerging field in America, and membership in the International Association of Yoga Therapists tripled from 2008 to 2011. Yoga therapists address specific health problems with specific postures, moves or poses, which change each week as the student progresses. Yoga has been used for managing high blood pressure, coping with the side effects of cancer treatment, alleviating symptoms of HIV, depression and anxiety, and relieving musculoskeletal issues like pain in the back, shoulder, neck and hip.

WHERE TO
GO FROM HERE

Now that you've seen the wealth of available holistic treatment options, you're probably wondering: What's next? Where do I go from here?

The answer is both simple and complex: Find whatever path is right for you. But the hard part is, you must do your homework and figure out, as Bob Seger sang, what to leave in and what to leave out. There is no single blueprint for everyone. Any given treatment may help with one disorder, but will perhaps ignore another. What is good for the body is not always good for the mind or the spirit, and vice versa.

You are a multidimensional, whole person, and you should be respected for your diversity. That's why you must find someone who will listen to your personal goals and be able to call upon the resources to help you realize them. This person—he or she could be an MD, a psychotherapist, or a focused professional like an acupuncturist—will serve as your health fusion coach and team leader.

One important caveat: Do not ask for or expect guarantees, and if someone offers you one, run away. Bernie Madoff couldn't provide the investment returns he touted without a Ponzi scheme, and if anything sounds too good to be true, it probably is.

Remember, the quest for better health is a natural process that does not always have a predictable outcome.

HOW TO FIND A HOLISTIC PRACTITIONER

By now, you understand that a holistic practitioner can be conventional or nonconventional, as long as that practitioner embraces a combination of both treatment options. He or she could be a medical doctor, psychotherapist, acupuncturist or any other kind of professional. When I started my journey, doctors David Padden and John Coats filled that role for me.

At International Holistic Center (IHC), which I founded in Fort Lauderdale, Florida, my practitioners and I serve our patients the same way. We help all patients build their own team to address their own needs. Your practitioners' specific disciplines do not matter, as long as they can see beyond their own horizons and help you find the best treatment options. That is truly being holistic.

Here are some tips:

1. Rely on word of mouth. Talk to friends who have used nonconventional treatments, or seek referrals from conventional doctors you trust.

2. Use a phone directory or go online to search headings such as integrative, alternative or nonconventional medicine. Or, zero in on the most promising—to you—individual types of treatment. For example, you might want to look at acupuncture or hypnotherapy.

3. Scan Internet referral lists, paying close attention to patient reviews. Keep in mind that I have seen great doctors who had a few poor reviews written by a few disgruntled patients. The Internet can make it too easy for people to disseminate false information.

4. Before you make an appointment for treatment, make an appointment for an interview. Go armed with written questions, and make sure they are answered. Get references. Ask

yourself this question: Is this person an ego-driven prima donna, or someone who wants to work in a partnership with you and lead your team? One red flag: If the practitioner says nothing about diet or nutrition, head for the door. This is true when you're dealing with conventional practitioners such as medical doctors: You should have the same standards for everyone who takes care of your health.

5. In addition to following up on references and credentials, check with the state for complaints and disciplinary action.

6. Check costs and insurance coverage. If, before the initial consultation, the practitioner wants to put you through expensive tests that are not covered by insurance, you may want to rethink the visit.

7. If you're dealing with an MD, check hospital privileges and find out who's on call when the doctor is unavailable. Is it another holistic practitioner, or is it someone who practices only conventional medicine?

THE HOLISTIC TEAM

A multidisciplinary-holistic approach is the best approach. Ideally, your team will give you access to a range of services. Here's one example of what a holistic team looks like:

*acupuncturist

*massage therapist

*psychotherapist

*anesthesiologist

*neurologist

*orthopedic surgeon

*oncologist

*nutritionist

*hypnotherapist

*nurse

*physical therapist

*occupational therapist

*social worker

*vocational counselor

I started the IHC because I wanted to provide clients with one-stop holistic treatment. If you can find a center or integrative practice that offers many different options under one roof, you won't have to run around trying to assemble your team yourself.

Be efficient—find a boutique center like IHC that has what you want and makes sense for you. Now remember what I said earlier in this book: Just because someone adds the word "wellness" or "holistic" to the name of a company, doesn't make it so.

Be educated, be informed, and don't give up.

Dr. Elizabeth King

RESOURCES

Alcoholics Anonymous
www.aa.org
P.O. Box 459
New York, NY 10163
212-870-3400
Mission: Recovery from alcoholism.

Alliance for Natural Health – USA (formerly American Association for Health Freedom)
www.anh-usa.org
1350 Connecticut Ave. NW, 5th Floor
Washington, DC 20036
800-230-2762
Mission: An international organization promoting sustainable health and freedom of choice in health care through science and law.

American Association of Acupuncture and Oriental Medicine
www.aaaomonline.org

9650 Rockville Pike
Bethesda, MD 20814
866-455-7999
Mission: To promote and advance high ethical, educational and professional standards in the practice of acupuncture and Oriental medicine in the United States.

American Association for the Advancement of Behavioral Therapy
www.aabt.org
Mission: Clearinghouse for links to psychological treatment providers and other resources.

American Association of Drugless Practitioners
www.aadp.net
2200 Market Street, Suite 803
Galveston, TX 77550-1530
409-621-2600
888-764-AADP
Mission: To promote equality between practitioners of conventional and nonconventional, or holistic, therapies.

American Cancer Society
www.cancer.org
250 Williams Street NW
Atlanta, GA, 30303
800-227-2345

Mission: To eliminate cancer as a major health problem by preventing cancer, saving lives and diminishing suffering from cancer, through research, education, advocacy and service.

American Chronic Pain Association
www.theacpa.org
P.O. Box 850
Rocklin, CA 95677
800-533-3231
E-mail: **acpa@pacbell.net**
Mission: Peer support and education in pain-management skills for people with pain, family and friends, and health care professionals.

American Headache Society Committee on Headache Education
www.achenet.org
Mission: Educational resource for patient-health professional partnerships, providing information materials, tools and resources that support both patients with disabling headaches and their families.

American Holistic Medical Association
www.holisticmedicine.org
27629 Chagrin Blvd., Suite 213
Woodmere, OH 44122
216-292-6644
e-mail: **info@holisticmedicine.org**

Mission: Professional and patient referrals to holistic practitioners.

American Holistic Nurses Association
www.ahna.org
323 N. San Francisco St., Suite 201
Flagstaff, AZ 86001
928-526-2196
800-278-2462
e-mail: info@ahna.org
Mission: To promote the education of nurses, other health care professionals, and the public in all aspects of holistic caring and healing.

American Pain Foundation
www.painfoundation.org
201 N. Charles St., Suite 710
Baltimore, MD 21201
888-615-PAIN (7246)
Mission: To educate, support and advocate for people affected by pain.

American Society of Alternative Therapists
www.asat.org
P.O. Box 303
Topsfield, MA 01983
978-561-1639
E-mail: asat@asat.org
Mission: To represent the professional and educational association of certified ASAT™ C.O.R.E. Counselors.

Anxiety Disorders Association of America
www.adaa.org
8730 Georgia Ave.
Silver Spring, MD 20910
240-485-1001
Mission: To promote the prevention, treatment, and cure of anxiety and stress-related disorders through advocacy, education, training, and research.

Arthritis Foundation
www.arthritis.org
P.O. Box 7669
Atlanta, GA 30357
800-283-7800
Mission: To help people take control of arthritis by providing public health education; pursuing public policy and legislation, and conducting evidence-based programs to improve the quality of life for those living with arthritis.

Association for Applied Psychophysiology and Biofeedback
www.aapb.org
10200 West 44th Ave. Suite 304
Wheat Ridge, CO 80033
303-422-8436
800-477-8892
E-mail: info@aapb.org

Mission: To advance the development, spread and use of knowledge about applied psychophysiology and biofeedback to improve health and the quality of life through research, education and practice.

Centers for Disease Control and Prevention
www.cdc.gov
1600 Clifton Rd.
Atlanta, GA 30333
800-CDC-INFO (232-4636)
E-mail: **cdcinfo@cdc.gov**
Mission: To collaborate with partners in the United States and the world to create the expertise, information, and tools that people and communities need to protect their health—through health promotion, prevention of disease, injury and disability, and preparedness for new health threats.

Coalition for Natural Health
www.healingfeats.com
1200 L Street N.W., Suite 100-408
Washington, DC 20005
800-586-4264
E-mail: info@naturalhealth.org
Mission: To provide legal protection to natural health consultants, holistic health practitioners, nutritional consultants, herbalists and others who wish to practice natural health exclusively.

EMDR International Association
www.emdria.org
5806 Mesa Drive, Suite 360
Austin, TX 78731
512-451-5200
866-451-5200
E-mail: **info@emdria.org**
Mission: A membership organization of mental health professionals dedicated to the highest standards of excellence and integrity in EMDR.

The Gladys T. McGarey Medical Foundation
www.mcgareyfoundation.org
4848 E. Cactus Rd., Suite 505-506
Scottsdale, AZ 85254
480-946-4544
Mission: To advance the cause of holistic medicine.

International Critical Incident Stress Foundation, Inc.
www.icisf.org
3290 Pine Orchard Lane, Suite 106
Ellicott City, MD 21042
410-750-9600
E-mail: info@icisf.org
Mission: To provide leadership, education, training, consultation and support for crisis intervention and disaster-behavioral-health services to the emergency-response professions, other organizations, and communities worldwide.

International Holistic Center
3471 North Federal Hwy, Ste 410
Fort Lauderdale, FL 33306
954-903-9426
CEO: Dr. Elizabeth King, LCSW
E-mail: DrKing@IHCHealthfusion.com
Website: www.IHCHealthfusion.com
Mission: To effectively fuse conventional and non-conventional assessments and treatments to address the problem at the core level, not just the symptoms.

The Mayday Pain Project
www.painandhealth.org
E-mail: maydaypain@aol.com
Mission: A purely educational Internet resource to help people improve self-management of their pain condition, written with the help of health educators, pain experts, and people dealing with pain.

Medline Plus
www.nlm.nih.gov/medlineplus
Mission: A service of the U.S. National Library of Medicine providing trusted health information for consumers.

Narcotics Anonymous
www.na.org
P.O. Box 9999
Van Nuys, CA 91409

818-773-9999
Mission: To recover from drug addiction.

National Association of Social Workers
www.socialworkers.org
750 First Street, N.E., Suite 700
Washington, D.C. 20002
202-408-8600
Mission: To enhance the professional growth and development of its social worker members, to create and maintain professional standards, and to advance sound social policies.

The National Center for PTSD (NCPTSD)
www.ncptsd.va.gov
Department of Veterans Affairs
800-827-1000
Mission: To advance science and to promote an understanding of post-traumatic stress disorder (PTSD).

National Center for Victims of Crime
www.ncvc.org
2000 M Street, N.W., Suite 480
Washington, D.C. 20036
202-467-8700
Mission: A resource and advocacy organization for crime victims and those who serve them.

National Coalition Against Domestic Violence

www.ncadv.org
One Broadway, Suite B210
Denver, CO 80203
303-839-1852
E-mail: mainoffice@ncadv.org
Mission: To organize for collective power by advancing transformative work, thinking and leadership of communities and individuals working to end violence against women and children.

National Headache Foundation
www.headaches.org
820 N. Orleans, Suite 411
Chicago, IL 60610
312-274-2650
888-NHF-5552
E-mail: info@headaches.org
Mission: To provide educational and informational resources, supports headache research, and advocates for the understanding of headache as a legitimate neurobiological disease—all to enhance the health care of individuals with headache.

National Institute of Dental and Craniofacial Research
www.nidcr.nih.gov
866-232-4528
e-mail: nidcrinfo@mail.nih.gov

Mission: To improve oral, dental and craniofacial health through research, research training, and the dissemination of health information.

National Institute on Drug Abuse
www.nida.nih.gov
6001 Executive Blvd.
Room 5213, MSC 9561
Bethesda, MD 20892
301-443-1124
E-mail: **information@nida.nih.gov**
Mission: To lead the nation in bringing the power of science to bear on drug abuse and addiction, through strategic support and performing research, and, by ensuring the rapid and effective dissemination and use of results of that research, to improve prevention and treatment and to inform policy as it relates to drug abuse and addiction.

National Institute of Mental Health (NIMH)
www.nimh.nih.gov
6001 Executive Blvd.
North Bethesda, MD 20852
301-443-4513
866-615-6464
E-mail: **nimhinfo@nih.gov**
Mission: To transform the understanding and treatment of mental illnesses through basic and clinical research, paving the way for prevention, recovery, and cure.

National Sexual Violence Resource Center
www.nsvrc.org
123 North Enola Dr.
Enola, PA 17025
717-909-0710
877-739-3895
E-mail: resources@nsvrc.org

Mission: To provide national leadership, consultation and technical assistance by generating and facilitating the development and flow of information on sexual violence intervention and prevention strategies, working to address the causes and impact of sexual violence through collaboration, prevention efforts, and the distribution of resources.

Ondamed®
www.Ondamed.net
Ondamed, Inc.
2570 Route 9W
Cornwall, NY 12518
845-534-0456
e-mail: support@ondamed.net

Mission: To educate medical professionals with scientific facts that are researched and published by leading scientists, particularly in regard to the Ondamed System, a physiological treatment that uses focused electromagnetic waves to stimulate improvement of systemic functions, as well as to improve stress-tolerance levels.

Rape, Abuse, and Incest National Network
www.rainn.org
2000 L Street, NW, Suite 406
Washington, DC 20036
202.544.3064
Hotline: 800-656-HOPE (4673)
Online hotline: rainn.org
E-mail: info@rainn.org
Mission: To operate confidential hotlines that educate the public about sexual violence and to lead national efforts to prevent sexual violence, improve services to victims, and ensure that rapists are brought to justice.

Young Living Essential Oils
www.youngliving.org/drkingnassoc
Dr. King and Associates PA
International Holistic Center
3471 N. Federal Hwy., Suite 410
Fort Lauderdale, FL 33306
954-903-9426
E-mail: **drking@ihchealthfusion.com**
Mission: To distribute essential oils for aromatherapy.

EMPOWERMENT MANTRA

Sometimes we need to remind ourselves of our own power and strength. When we are in physical or emotional pain, it is even more challenging to be assertive and to feel good about ourselves and clear about our rights.

This empowerment mantra will help you begin your day with the necessary self-talk for effective change. Indulge. This is your time for healing.

Please repeat the following statements every morning and as often as you need to reinforce your commitment to getting better. Do it sitting or lying down in a quiet room. Before you begin, please take a deep lung-filled breath. Inhale through your nose and exhale slowly through your mouth. Allow yourself a few minutes to internalize the words after you read them aloud.

Today...I am strong. I will not allow my condition to consume me.

Today...I am ready to be proactive and take control of my life.

Today...I am in charge of my life.

Today...I am in charge of my medical treatment.

Today...I will not be intimidated by any health care professional.

Today...I will not be discouraged.

Today...I will demand holistic and comprehensive quality care.

Today...I am entitled to understand my treatment options.

Today...I understand that knowledge is power. I will read, research, and apply what I learn about my mind and my body.

Today...I choose to have a high quality of life.

Today...I choose to be happy.

DR. KING'S PERSONAL TIPS FOR STAYING YOUNG AND AGING HEALTHIER

Every day of our lives, whether we think about it or not, we use tricks drawn from our own experience that have become so engrained, we think of them as habits.

This list of tricks, or shortcuts, is yours for the taking. They are all about living well and growing older gracefully.

Add items from your own list, and have fun. As the great comedian (and philosopher) Lucille Ball said,

"The secret to staying young is to live honestly, eat slowly, and lie about your age."

1. Drink half your weight in ounces of water every day. For example, if you weigh 150 pounds, you should drink 75 ounces of water per day. Divide that by 8 ounces per glass, and you have 9 glasses of water per day.

2. Put a drop of Young Living™ lemon essential oil in each glass of water to purify it. Unless your water is filtered, it may have a high concentration of impurities.

3. Try not to use microwaves, but if you must use them, don't warm up food in plastic containers.

4. Use a natural, low-glycemic sweetener such as organic blue agave nectar, grade B maple syrup, fructose or stevia. Do not use the sweeteners that come in pink, yellow, blue, brown or white packages.

5. Maintain your body's alkalinity: Test your pH at least once a month. Eat lemons, garlic, yellow and green veggies, beans and whole nuts. Avoid overuse of antibiotics. Use essential oils, which contain antibacterial and antifungal properties. Clove and thyme kill 15 different strains of fungi. Use alkaline minerals, which lower stress. Boost friendly flora, or, beneficial bacteria, by adding acidophilus supplements and yogurt to your diet.

6. Don't use skin or hair products containing the widely used preservatives called parabens.

7. Don't use deodorants containing aluminum.

8. Do a colon cleanse regularly to rid your body of internal debris. You can do it at home or at a hydro-colonics center. Some essential oils and coffee enemas are effective for this as well.

9. Eat organic, hormone-free meats and eggs and fish caught in the wild.

10. Don't skip breakfast. Eat or drink proteins in the morning. Have carbs for lunch. Have fruits and vegetables and a small amount of protein for dinner.

11. Don't eat after 7 p.m. If you must eat after 7 p.m., avoid starches and sugary fruits.

12. Move your body every day. Walk, exercise, dance, jog, bike, or swim. Get your heart rate up and keep it there for at least 20 minutes. Exercise with 5-10 pound weights to maintain muscle tone.

13. Massage your face daily. To help eliminate the toxins in your body, reduce stress and stimulate healthy cellular growth, schedule therapeutic massages at least once a month—more if you have a chronic condition.

14. Take daily supplements: Juice Plus™ (in fruit, vegetable and berry capsules), Vitamins C, E and D, and omega oils. Other supplements target specific chronic conditions.

15. Try to sleep seven to eight hours every night. I personally need just five hours of sleep to feel rested, but I get up and spend time meditating before I begin my day. To help you get to sleep, use lavender or Peace and Calming™ on the bottom of your feet, under your nose and on your pillow. Mix it with water and spray it in your room. Drink chamomile tea one hour before bedtime.

16. Go for acupuncture every three months to promote well-being. Go more often if you suffer from a physical condition that acupuncture treats.

17. Have your hormones checked annually and, if hormone replacement is needed, seek the natural kind.

18. Use fluoride-free toothpaste.

19. Spend time with positive people.

20. Meditate and pray.

21. Laugh at least twice a day. If you can manage a belly laugh, that's even better.

22. Live in gratitude. Pay it forward. And have fun as often as you can!

Recipe for Creating Your Happiest Life

One of the most famous phrases ever written is from the Declaration of Independence: "life, liberty and the pursuit of happiness."

It doesn't matter what socio-economic background you come from, where you were born, or what you want to do in life—simply put, we are all pursuing happiness. Mind you, "happiness" is a very personal emotion. If you ask a hundred people to define happiness, you will have a hundred different definitions.

Nevertheless, we are all trying to live our happiest life. On the surface, achieving happiness appears to be a simple task, but actually it is a very complex process that requires commitment, hard work and perseverance.

So why stress ourselves in pursuit of happiness if it is going to take so much out of us? Because the rewards are as sweet as eating a warm piece of double chocolate cake with a scoop of creamy vanilla bean ice cream (organic, of course).

I am not going to bore you with a detailed description of the biology of feeling happy. But I promise you the endorphin high that you feel when you are happiest is well worth the work it took to get there.

Maybe a cynic would say that people can achieve happiness without the hard work, just by altering their minds with substances like drugs or alcohol. The problem with that theory is this type of happiness is only temporary, and always short-lived.

Living your happiest life means having inner peace, so any feeling of euphoria that doesn't foster inner peace is not true happiness.

After blank-blank years of life (yes, I am old enough to avoid sharing my age in print) and thirty years of studying the human mind, I think I have finally come up with the perfect recipe for creating your happiest life.

The great part of this recipe is that I get to share it with you and you get to make it your own. Staying true to my Latin heritage, I am not listing exact amounts of any of the ingredients because you need to put in "a little bit of this" and "a little bit of that" and "season to taste."

Ingredients:

Live with purpose

Remember that attitude is everything

Have gratitude

Spend time with positive people

Practice healthy living

Give back and pay it forward

Demonstrate patience

Make time for self-care

Create financial stability

Foster respectful relationships

Be spiritual (not necessarily religious)

Get enough rest

Do things you enjoy—often

Forgive quickly

Set appropriate boundaries

Strive for balance

Directions:

In the morning as soon as you wake up, take time
to consciously reflect on the list of ingredients listed

above. Take great care in making sure to have a clean table and utensils to begin preparing (open your mind to the possibilities and focus on your strengths). Wash down any leftovers from your mixing bowls (let go of your past). Pre-measure your ingredients and set them aside.

Get ready for mixing (be mindful of what you need to do). If you don't have all of the ingredients, figure out how to compensate (find ways to overcome your weaknesses). If you need help, ask an expert (don't be afraid to seek counseling or coaching).

Slowly blend an unlimited amount of the ingredients, adjusting to taste (happiness is in the eye of the beholder, so let inner peace guide you). Blend at a moderate speed until you can't see any separation (it all comes together seamlessly). Drizzle with forgiveness and sprinkle with some more patience.

You are ready to serve. If you did it well, you will have a smooth and creamy consistency. The taste will be decadent and sweet.

This recipe makes enough to feed your soul and give you inner peace (you will even have leftovers to be consumed during hard times). If it doesn't come out the way you like it (if you are not living your happiest life), don't give up, but start again. This time, sprinkle some more "giving back" and "forgiveness," and double the "balance" and "fun" (in my experience these are usually the missing ingredients).

For best results, let it marinate. Now go ahead and savor your creation!

How to Deal with Chronic Pain without Taking Drugs

I am an expert on chronic pain—not only because in my practice I treat patients suffering from it, but because excruciating pain plagued me for years, until I was able to control and overcome it by using a combination of holistic treatments.

There was a time not terribly long ago when I had to struggle to get out of bed and walk with a walker. A veteran of thirty-five operations stemming from childhood polio, I plummeted to the depths of a pain-filled hell through a simple fall from an elevator that tore the meniscus disc in my knee. Of course, the torn meniscus was just the final straw after two hip replacements within four years.

After two years of taking painkillers and depending on others to help me get around and to accomplish the simplest of tasks, I was actually reduced to hoping a doctor would find the cancerous tumor I was certain was growing in my body—just so I would have an answer and maybe a path to recovery.

Fortunately, I did not have cancer. That visit to a specialist changed my life. It led to my first tentative contact with acupuncture and the rest of the world of nonconventional treatments.

If you are like I was, you are searching for alternative approaches to deal with chronic pain. You are seeking methods that do not involve drugs because they can become addictive and further burden your life.

Here is my advice, the product of my own experience and of my patients at the IHC.

I have outlined several alternative techniques that will help you not only handle chronic pain, but improve the quality of your life.

Follow these approaches, which are healthy for your body and, even better, totally free of charge. These techniques are helpful in controlling migraines, muscular and arthritic tissue pain, internal bodily pain and pain in general.

1. Don't give in to your pain. No matter how severe the pain gets, don't let it control you. It's all about mind over matter. Your inner strength is there; tap into it. Soon you'll realize how powerful you are.

2. Breathe and visualize. Imagine being in a beautiful place like a seashore, walking in the mountains, or sitting on a couch by a fireplace in the middle of a thunderstorm. Take deeps breaths, in through your nose and out through your mouth. Use all of your senses to put yourself there. Try to experience the sounds and smells of that particular environment. Do this anytime your pain flares up or just do it when you feel like taking a mini-vacation. You'll soon get so good that you'll feel the ocean breeze and smell the salt water.

3. Make facial expressions and loosen up your face and jaw. Stretch your facial muscles by opening your mouth as wide as you can. Hold it for a minute or two. The feeling will be a bit uncomfortable, but just hang in there. When you feel the muscles in your jaw and head pulling and tingling, relax. This will probably be very painful momentarily and make your eyes water, but it helps tremendously with the pain over time.

4. Use your hands. Be your own massage therapist. Apply pressure to your trigger points. Use your second and third digits to rub softly in a circular motion. This is also helpful when applied to painful organs.

Massage the trigger points on the collarbone, the back of the head or wherever they may be for you. Sometimes it is more effective to use the thumb for deep penetration into areas such as the collarbone. Gently press the trigger points until it feels like you will go through the ceiling and your eyes tear. Then go ahead and release the pressure. Do this several times to each painful or tender area.

5. Loosen muscles with a hot shower. Get into a steamy bath with the water as hot as you can bear it. Put the painful area under the hot water for fifteen minutes. Keep the steam in the room by closing all the windows and the door. You can also use some of the other techniques, such as the breathing method and trigger-point massage, while you are in the shower.

6. Spend time with loved ones who have a positive outlook on life. It is important to surround yourself with people who exude positive energy, mainly because this type of optimistic exchange will help your mind and body feel at ease. And who better to connect with than your closest relatives? Have light-hearted conversations, share jokes, play cards or just sit and enjoy silent company. Their radiance will help you heal.

7. Exercise. Believe it or not, exercise is the best stress release available. If you reduce stress, you reduce pain.

8. Close your eyes and enjoy your own world. This is probably the most enjoyable technique because you get to sleep and/or meditate. Lie down, close your eyes and focus on the area that is causing you pain. Picture a ball of light revolving around the area. Bring that healing light all around your body. Also, use the breathing technique to help you relax and release stress.

9. Feed your inner being. Participate in activities that make you happy: walking in the woods, keeping a journal, playing tennis, swimming in the ocean, reading a book by the river, etc. These little things are what nurture your soul.

10. Express your pain verbally. An excellent way to deal with pain is to speak with someone who is empathetic. It's very unhealthy to keep whatever is bothering you bottled up. Tell someone understanding and compassionate about how awful it is and what it feels like. Vent, vent, vent.

If you don't want to verbalize out loud, then free-associate. Get a pen and paper and write down everything that comes to mind without editing yourself mentally. After you are done venting, close your eyes and practice your breathing technique, meditate, or listen to music. It is important to give yourself permission to have a "pity party" every so often, but make sure you don't get stuck in it. Set the timer and when the timer goes off, stop the party.

11. Seek the help of holistic pain professionals. Now that you have read my book, you have a better understanding of what holistic means and, I hope, more open to trying new therapies such as acupuncture, hypnosis, Ondamed®, or the type of nutritional counseling that targets foods that create inflammation. Literally hundreds of therapies treat pain effectively and are alternatives to medication or surgery.

A "(W)Holistic" Approach to Treating Depression

I wanted to write this because so many of my clients come to the IHC with symptoms of depression and say, "Dr. King, I think I need medication. I am depressed."

Worse still are the many clients who come in with their drugs already in hand, telling me that doctors put them on anti-depressants just because the patients said the magic word: "depression."

Many of my clients tell me they are put on anti-depressants after only five to ten minutes of meeting with a new doctor. Most of the time the doctor never even asks what is going on in the patient's life. The doctor just pulls out a prescription pad, writes out a prescription, and sends the patient on his or her way.

In one particular case, if the doctor had asked my client, she would have told him she had just lost her brother in a very bad car accident, she had lost her dog three weeks earlier, and her best friend had committed suicide a year before. She was also waiting for the results of a liver biopsy. No wonder she was experiencing symptoms of depression such as crying excessively, feeling overwhelmed and losing her appetite.

I would like to believe that was a rare case.

I am not saying the doctor was wrong to put her on an anti-depressant (I don't want to second-guess anyone). But there were so many other treatment options that should have been explored before jumping into medication.

Unfortunately in Western medicine, medication appears to be the cornerstone of how we treat everything. This concerns me greatly, and it should concern you, too. If you are one of those people who put all their faith in medication—like my client who said she "didn't believe in doing things naturally," she believed only in medication—please take a moment and hear what I am saying: Medication is not the only answer!!!

We all know that drugs may fix one problem but create ten other problems. If you don't believe me, just read the long list of possible side effects spelled out on the side of each prescription drug package. Now tell me why that doesn't worry you. Better yet, pay close attention to the ads on TV for prescription drugs and see how many possible side effects they spout off at the end of the commercial.

Don't get me wrong. I believe that prescribing medication is appropriate at times, as long as it is not the first reaction to any condition, especially depression.

Before you get on an anti-depressant, please read this!

I love putting a "w" before the word "holistic" because it makes the concept easier to understand. (W)holistic is the total or whole approach. In the context of health, it refers to the fusion of conventional and nonconventional methods of assessing and treating the whole person.

In my experience, a "(w)holistic" approach—including traditional psychiatry, pharmacology in some limited cases, and other options—offers better symptom resolution and long-term recovery than any single effort. The reason is that you are addressing the problem at the core level, not just the symptoms. An integrative health care practitioner or (w)holistic counselor will fully evaluate your history and physical condition and will coordinate your care to meet your individual needs.

If you do wind up needing an anti-depressant, the goal should be to wean yourself off it as soon as possible. Here are some options to explore before you even consider getting on an anti-depressant in the first place:

- Counseling—Talk therapy / EMDR / Cognitive-Behavioral therapy

- Hypnotherapy

- Ondamed® or another pulsed electro-magnetic field (PEMF) device

- Biofeedback

- Body work methods, such as therapeutic massage, Healing Touch, cranial-sacral therapy (CST) and acupuncture

- Oriental medicinal herbs

- Nutritional counseling and supplements such as fruit and vegetable capsules, vitamins, minerals and omega-3 fatty acids

- Aromatherapy

- Meditation

- Exercise such as yoga

Treat your depression—naturally

I hope that after you read this article, it makes perfect sense to you that the first thing you should try is treating your depression naturally. After all, medications will always be there if you absolutely need them.

Now, that doesn't mean you need to do anything alone. A wide range of holistic health care providers will support you if you choose to go this route. Start off with a holistic psychotherapist who will guide you through the process.

There may be some comfort in knowing that depression offers us a reason to examine and change our lives. Think about how your circumstances may be affecting your outlook. Make sure you think about what you eat and when you eat—this can have a big impact on your mood. Pay close attention to your sleep patterns, your environment, the way you spend your time, and with whom you spend it. And don't be afraid to try something new.

Explore your spirituality. How do you make sense of the world? Join a support group that focuses on setting goals. Listen to music. Make time to listen to a motivational message every day. Be kind to yourself; take some time to find what feels good and right for you. And don't be afraid to ask for a helping hand.

It may be hard to believe now, but feeling down is most likely temporary—time may be the kindest and gentlest healer of all. And you can rest assured knowing there are plenty of natural ways to support your mood and outlook along the way.

With some deep reflection, supportive guidance and hope, you can feel good again—in body, mind, and spirit. The important message is this: Never give up.

The ABCs of EMDR

Have you ever heard of EMDR? If you haven't, and you or someone you love suffers from symptoms of post-traumatic stress disorder (PTSD), anxiety, depression, panic attacks or chronic pain, you need to find out whether EMDR can help.

Research has shown that EMDR is effective. As a therapist who uses EMDR almost daily in my practice, I can tell you that I have seen incredible results.

For those readers who are skeptical because you have tried all sorts of therapies and little or nothing has worked, ask yourself, "What do I have to lose?" EMDR may change your life or the life of a loved one.

What does EMDR stand for and who developed it?

EMDR stands for Eye Movement Desensitization and Reprocessing. It was developed in 1987 by a psychologist, Dr. Francine Shapiro. In 1989, Dr. Shapiro published encouraging results of EMDR therapy for the treatment of PTSD in the *Journal of Traumatic Stress* and won recognition for her work.

For more than twenty years, practitioners have been busy applying this technique and achieving un-believable results. Today EMDR therapy is widely used and accepted worldwide for treating trauma and many other conditions.

How and why does EMDR work?

Quite honestly, even researchers have a difficult time ex-plaining how and why EMDR works. At some level it is still a bit of a mystery. But regardless of its complexity, the end result is, it has been proven to work. As a trained EMDR therapist who uses it continually, I agree that EMDR is very effective, especially when combined with other treatments that address problems at the core level.

In EMDR, the client focuses on a disturbing image or event. Meanwhile the therapist facilitates a rapid, bilateral (left to right) eye movement that allows the brain to reprocess and neutralize the emotion attached to the image or event. Typically it takes three to eight EMDR sessions to achieve successful results.

What happens when you experience a traumatic event?

When you experience a traumatic event, your brain goes into the flight-or-fight mode to protect you. If the experience is too intense or overwhelming, or if you are traumatized repeatedly, your brain may go into a "freeze" mode because it can't process the experience and let it go.

Young children are especially impacted by extreme situations. They just don't have the neurobiological capability (fight or flight) or the coping skills to help them neutralize an actual or perceived life-threatening situation.

An adult may also go into a freeze mode upon experiencing a traumatic situation such as a car accident, a threatened assault with a gun, or a rape. Other events that may appear on the surface not to be as traumatic—like someone who is afraid of snakes being confronted by one in the backyard, or a child getting bullied at school—can also send the brain into a freeze mode.

The outcome is devastating because the moment gets frozen in time, to the point that remembering the event may bring back smells, sounds, feelings and images as if it were happening for the first time.

According to EMDRIA, the certifying body for EMDR therapists, EMDR appears to have a direct effect on the way the brain processes information. After EMDR therapy, the person finds that he or she no longer relives the traumatic experience. Nor does the person have the intense emotions attached to the memory of the event.

What kind of problems can EMDR treat?

Research has proven that EMDR is a highly effective method of psychotherapy for treating PTSD. EMDR reportedly has also been successful in the treatment of other conditions such as pain disorders, panic attacks, complicated grief, dissociative disorders, depression, disturbing memories, phobias, addictions, perform-ance anxiety, stress, sexual and/or physical abuse, and body dysmorphic and eating disorders.

I do not have empirical data to prove this, but I believe EMDR works for many of those conditions because if you peel the onion down far enough, you will find the condition was triggered by a traumatic event.

For example, if someone is suffering from panic attacks, I would develop a timeline of events to try to determine whether the person was traumatized and is still in the freeze mode. Often there is quite a bit of unresolved or unacknowledged trauma. Finding the original trauma creates a perfect scenario to begin EMDR therapy.

How do I know if EMDR is right for me?

EMDR is not magical and it certainly is not right for everyone. Yet EMDR is a neuropsychological approach that has helped many people, so I recommend you at least explore it.

A trained EMDR therapist will conduct a thorough evaluation and consider a number of factors when deciding whether the therapy is right for you. Make sure to educate yourself before starting EMDR so you understand the pros and cons. A good therapist will welcome your questions and help you decide whether you should proceed with this treatment protocol.

Don't be afraid to try EMDR if your therapist recommends it. Therapists who are qualified to use EMDR go through rigorous training before they are allowed to incorporate it into their practices.

How do I find a trained EMDR therapist?

Most therapists who are trained in EMDR will list their training as part of their credentials on their business cards, websites and promotional materials.

Go to www.EMDRIA.org. You can use the website to locate an EMDR therapist in your area.

Ask your friends and family for a recommendation. EMDR therapy has become quite popular in the past decade, and since many people have learned how effective it is, they probably know of a qualified EMDR therapist.

Finally, ask your therapist if she or he is EMDR trained. Sometimes we forget to inform our clients/ patients of all the things we are trained to do. This actually happened to one of my colleagues.

Bark like a Dog or Quack like a Duck: The Facts and Fiction about Hypnosis

I decided to write this because it dawned on me that there are still a lot of misconceptions about what hypnosis is, and what it isn't.

Few days go by at my IHC when I don't hear from a new client the infamous question: "If you hypnotize me, are you going to make me bark like a dog or quack like a duck?" The clients always chuckle nervously after asking the question, as if to say, "I really don't believe in hypnosis."

Well, don't feel embarrassed if you're one of those people who have asked that same question (even if only to yourself). I must admit I was guilty of asking the question before discovering I needed to learn about hypnosis (see page 1 to read about my journey with chronic pain and how hypnotherapy helped get me back on my feet).

I don't want to make excuses for all of us who have experienced doubts about hypnosis, but our perception of it might have been formulated by watching stage performers at a comedy club, for example. Their job was to make us all laugh about the silly commands they called out to participants who were "willing to make themselves look foolish." All in the name of fun. Of course, most of us left the comedy club saying, "There is no way that was real."

If you have been exposed to the research on the many uses of hypnotherapy, you are ahead of the game and probably chuckling right now at how naive this sounds. Unfortunately for many of us, we learn how effective hypnosis can be because we have tried everything else, and hypnosis becomes our last resort and only hope for getting relief from whatever ails us.

Sparked by headlines about celebrities overdosing, there has been a lot more interest recently in finding creative ways to avoid drugs and alleviate the problems associated with living in the limelight. One of those ways is hypnosis. Mainstream medical journals and TV shows like "Good Morning America" and "Prime Time Live" have highlighted hypnosis as a

viable option for relieving the symptoms of psychological and physiological conditions.

As more people become educated about hypnosis,
I foresee that "traditional" medical practitioners will
be forced to incorporate it into their clinical practices.

**What are the misconceptions and facts about
hypnosis?**

I know there are a whole lot more misconceptions
about hypnosis than the ones I am listing here. But
if I can clarify some of the more common ones, then
maybe some of you doubters will be willing to research whether hypnosis is right for you. I hope this
helps.

Misconception: Hypnosis is a sham.

Fact: Many top health care professionals are using
hypnosis as part of their treatment protocol and seeing
great results in their patients. Simply put, hypnosis
uses the power of the mind to overcome barriers and
achieve positive changes.

**Misconception: For hypnosis to work, the subject
must be gullible.**

Fact: Research has shown that most people can
benefit from hypnosis. Choosing to be responsive to
suggestion means you understand the concept of how

hypnosis works and are willing to allow your mind and body to do what is natural. In my practice, I have not noticed IQ to be at all reflective of a client's ability to be hypnotized.

Misconception: The person being hypnotized is under the control of the hypnotist and can be made to do or say anything the hypnotist wants.

Fact: No matter how deeply hypnotized you are, you remain in total control. You cannot be made to do anything you do not want to do. Rest assured that no one can make you bark like a dog or quack like a duck unless you agree to do it.

Misconception: Hypnosis is done to someone else, rather than to oneself.

Fact: Hypnosis is a skill you can learn. It is a tool you can use to help yourself feel better. My own experience with self-hypnosis magnified the effects of acupuncture and massage and helped alleviate the chronic pain that had virtually incapacitated me for two years.

Misconception: You can be trapped in hypnosis and may never come out of it.

Fact: You may end hypnosis whenever you want. Just as you cannot stay asleep forever, you cannot be under hypnosis forever.

Misconception: During hypnosis, you are unconscious or asleep.

Fact: During hypnosis, you are not asleep or unconscious. You are just in a deep state of relaxation. Although many of my clients do fall asleep because they feel very relaxed, they are still aware of everything and are active participants in the process.

Misconception: You have to be lying down in a quiet place to be able to enter a hypnotic trance.

Fact: You can go into a hypnotic trance sitting up or lying down. It is all about practicing to be tuned into your mind and body. An experienced hypnotherapist can teach you how to do self-hypnosis anywhere.

What is hypnosis used for?

The Mayo Clinic reports that hypnotherapy can be used to:

- Reduce or eliminate anxiety, phobias or depression

- Change negative behaviors such as smoking, overeating or addictions

- Lower blood pressure

- Control pain from injury or chronic illness, surgery or childbirth

- Reduce the intensity or frequency of migraines

- Help heal skin diseases, including warts and psoriasis

Based on my own experience, hypnotherapy can also be used to:

- Lose weight

- Improve self-esteem and reach your highest potential

- Enhance athletic and business performance

- Relieve stress

How can I choose a great hypnotherapist?

The answer is simple: Research a hypnotherapist's credentials such as certification, ask around for references, and, most importantly, schedule an appointment to ask lots of questions. Having a good rapport with the hypnotherapist, feeling that she or he is knowledgeable, and understanding the process are crucial to enabling you to relax enough to be guided into hypnosis.

Depending on where you live, researching a professional hypnotherapist's licensing may be another avenue to finding a practitioner. Make sure that the license of the person you're researching is active, and that there has been no serious disciplinary action against that person.

Because Florida, where I live and work, does not require hypnotherapists to be licensed, anyone can hang out a shingle, so other forms of vetting become even more important. Fortunately, many highly qualified and licensed mental health professionals are also certified hypnotherapists.

And remember: Hypnosis works only if you are *really* ready to embrace change. Hypnosis is not magic, but it is effective!

YOUR CHECKLIST

Here are some questions you'll want to have handy when you talk to a prospective holistic practitioner:

1. How do you define your practice?

2. After listening to my symptoms and problems, what treatment option or options would you recommend for me?

3. What is your recommendation based on?

4. Have you treated people with my condition before? If so, what were the results?

5. Are there any conventional or alternative types of treatments that you wouldn't recommend for anyone? If so, why?

6. Would you be willing to work as part of a team with me and my other health care providers?

7. (If the practitioner has received poor patient reviews.) Can you respond to these bad reviews?

8. (If the practitioner has been the subject of disciplinary action.) Can you explain this disciplinary action?

9. What are your references and credentials?

10. Do you believe that diet and nutrition are important aspects of holistic health care?

11. What is your policy on testing?

12. Who would I see if you were unavailable? Do you have a back-up who shares your treatment philosophy?

13. Do you guarantee good results? (If the answer is yes, head for the nearest exit. Neither allopathic doctors nor holistic practitioners should be offering guarantees because you are a human being, not a machine with standard parts.)

YOUR INFORMATION

Feel free to copy this form and complete it before you go to see a practitioner. It will save you a lot of time if you gather your information before you go to your appointment. Use multiple forms if needed.

I. INSURANCE INFORMATION (if applicable):

Most practitioners need a copy of your insurance card (front and back) and driver's license. Please bring them with you.

Insurance Company Name: _____

_____

Insurance ID Number: _____

Group Number: _____

II. MENTAL HEALTH HISTORY:

Previous psychiatric/substance abuse treatment: (include reason for treatment and dates)

Be specific.

III. MEDICAL HISTORY (including chronic illness-es, surgeries, injuries, allergies and communicable diseases):

Name of Primary Care Doctor:_____

Address:_____

City:_____

Phone #: _____

State:_____ Zip Code:_____

IV. MEDICATION: List them all, including dosages.

PRESCRIBING PHYSICIAN:

Specific condition

Dates and duration

V. PLEASE LIST ALL HERBS, VITAMINS, AND NUTRITIONAL SUPPLEMENTS YOU ARE TAKING:

_____

_____

_____

_____

VI. PLEASE LIST ANY ALLERGIES OR SENSITIVITIES TO MEDICATION THAT YOU HAVE:

Dr. Elizabeth King

"Note Pages"

_____
_____
_____
_____
_____
_____
_____
_____
_____
_____
_____
_____
_____
_____
_____
_____
_____
_____
_____
_____
_____
_____
_____
_____
_____
_____
_____
_____

Dr. Elizabeth King

"Note Pages"

_____
_____
_____
_____
_____
_____
_____
_____
_____
_____
_____
_____
_____
_____
_____
_____
_____
_____
_____
_____
_____
_____
_____
_____
_____
_____
_____
_____
_____
_____

"Note Pages"

Dr. Elizabeth King

"Note Pages"

"Note Pages"

_____
_____
_____
_____
_____
_____
_____
_____
_____
_____
_____
_____
_____
_____
_____
_____
_____
_____
_____
_____
_____
_____
_____
_____
_____
_____
_____
_____
_____

Author's Biography

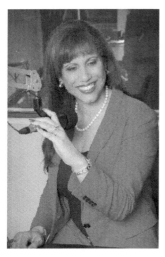

Dr. Elizabeth King is the CEO and founder of International Holistic Center (IHC) in Fort Lauderdale, Florida. She is an internationally renowned wellness expert, psychotherapist, corporate development leader, empowerment speaker, radio personality, coach and trainer. Dr. King also serves as an adjunct professor at Nova Southeastern University. She is regarded by her peers as a leader and a visionary.

Dr. King spent almost twenty years with the Broward County public school system, where she rose from teacher to administrator overseeing thirty programs and speaking nationally on behalf of children.

She founded the IHC with the goal of creating a center where nonconventional and conventional practitioners work together to treat and heal the whole person.

What started off as a dream is now a first-class holistic center that attracts people from around the globe. Using her impeccable leadership skills, Dr. King has put together a strong and dedicated—and growing—team of professionals who have helped her lead IHC to the highest tier of the health and wellness industry. IHC's revenues have almost quadrupled in the past two years and the center will expand to a space almost twice as big by fall 2012.

Currently, she is passionately coordinating her brainchild: the first-annual Women's International Holistic Conference. This global initiative will empower and inspire women to take control of their lives. Dr. King's next goal is to build the first holistic "hospital" in the country within eight to ten years.

In conjunction with running the center, Dr. King creates, produces and directs the highly acclaimed

"Dr. King's Health Fusion Hour," a weekly segment on AM radio. This show is dedicated to educating, inspiring, and empowering listeners to take full control of their health and lives. Her list of celebrated guests includes: Dr. Bernie Siegel, Mark Sanborn, Dr. Gladys McGarey, Dr. Robert DeMaria, Dr. Thomas Levy, Nina Hart, and other experts and authors in the holistic health field.

Dr. King has appeared on countless media outlets. She was also featured among the "100 most inspirational and motivational people" in Nina Hart's best-selling book, *Forever Young*.

Recently, Dr. King was selected for the Hispanic Women of Distinction Award 2012, a very prestigious honor. Also, she was nominated for the 2010 National Association of Women Business Owners Bravo Diversity Award.

Audiences connect immediately with Dr. King, not only because of her extensive clinical and leadership background, but because she speaks from the heart and has an infectious passion for helping people. Her captivating personal stories, combined with her knowledgeable remarks, always leave her audiences motivated, empowered and inspired to reach their highest potential. Dr. King speaks on topics ranging from wellness to leadership, increasing the bottom line, team-building, and work-life balance.

Dr. King has presented and delivered keynote speeches to countless organizations, corporations, colleges and universities. Here is an abbreviated list of the prestigious groups Dr. King has addressed: American Express, Women's Business Development Council of Florida, Ana Mendez University, Heart Camp, Aspira, Hogar Crea–Dominican Republic, Broward College, Pinellas County Schools, Pace Center for Girls, PR–Hispanic Chamber of Commerce, Team of Life, Red Hat Society–Salsera Fort Lauderdale chapter, National Association of Business Owners, South Florida Society for Trauma–Based Disorders, and the Rotary Club.

Dr. King earned her doctoral degree in educational leadership from Nova Southeastern University and her master's degree in social work from Florida International University. She has completed extensive post–graduate training in health and wellness, leadership and business development.

To receive Dr. King's Newsletter:

www.DrElizabethKing.com

www.IHChealthFusion.com

Stay connected:

Email: DrKing@IHCHealthFusion.com

Facebook : DrElizabethKing

Twitter: DrElizabethKing

Twitter: IHC_Broward

TESTIMONIALS

About Dr. Elizabeth King and the International Holistic Center:

"We had never had prior experience with holistic treatments. However, after 14 major surgeries and over 4 years of hospitalizations for my daughter, we were willing to try anything. Traditional medical treatments for my daughter kept her drugged to the point of being catatonic and at one point, landed her in a coma. The work that Dr. Elizabeth King and her team did with my daughter was life-changing and took us both by surprise. At this time, my daughter is much healthier and happier, as am I. However, the most important work the doctors do at the center is in how they care for their patients and they extended that level of caring to me at the lowest time in our lives. I highly recommend their holistic center to anyone in need of a better way of life."

C. & M.G.

"I went to see Dr. King when I was at the end of my rope. I had tried three other therapists that I did not connect with. I put a call in to her and within 15 minutes we had scheduled an appointment.

Dr. King was very open about how long it would take and what type of things we would be doing to cure my acute anxiety. It turns out that the symptoms I was feeling were from seeing domestic violence as a child, I guess a post-traumatic disorder. As far-fetched as I thought that was, I was wrong.

After a couple of visits Dr. King and I did EMDR therapy and after that first session, I had a heightened sense of anxiety, which apparently is normal. After a few days, that seemed to lessen, until I was completely calm. Once I was able to function in a calmer capacity, I was able to process things better.

The one thing that impressed me the most is that Dr. King does not push meds, she pushes therapy and gives you homework. I have completed my homework and my ongoing therapy. For the first time in over a year I am at peace. No more demons taking over my thoughts and causing the panic that once consumed me.

I believe in what she does so much that something that I would consider a taboo subject I have been discussing with my friends. I have suggested they also see Dr. King. Some have!

Thank you so much for all that you have done to return me to the person I was!"

W. W.

"Since I have been coming to IHC I am more focused. I have less anxiety, a better self-image, and a positive outlook.

The Center provides a relaxing environment as soon as you come through the door. Dr. King is a very compassionate, sincere, understanding person and pays attention to everything you say. Her relaxation/hypnosis is like getting a brain massage."

S. S.

"Dr. Elizabeth King has truly been an instrumental figure in my life, and she has served as a beacon of positive energy for me and my entire family. She has been a teacher, mentor, and advisor to me throughout my journey towards peace, tranquility and happiness. Although my journey has been challenging, Dr. King has been by my side to provide me with valuable insight. Her ability to relate to me through her own life experiences and challenges really makes her one of a kind. I would like to thank Dr. Elizabeth King for empowering me and helping change my life for the better."

A. A.

ACKNOWLEDGEMENTS

This is probably the most difficult section for me to write because I am so very grateful for the blessing of having a multitude of wonderful people in my life. Some have been involved directly in supporting me through the daunting task of writing this book while trying to run a center, see patients, produce a radio show, develop a lipstick line and present a conference. Others have been there throughout my life journey and without them, I know there would be no "Dr. Elizabeth King" and certainly this book would never have happened.

I have come to the conclusion that when you don't have legs to walk with, you grow wings to fly. The people listed here, along with so many more, have been my wings.

My gratitude goes to my extraordinary editor, Noreen Marcus, for being a "type A" personality. I had never met anyone as driven as me until I met her. I love that she is meticulous, a perfectionist and, at times, a task master, because without her I would never have met the many deadlines to get this book finished in time for my conference. She has given up many weekends and late evenings to help me meet deadlines and process thoughts, meanwhile providing words of encouragement. Her ability to see my vision and convert it into words is the reason this book is finally a reality. Through this process I have come to consider her a friend.

A special thank you to her husband, retired editor Joe Modzelewski, who has provided very meaningful feedback and lots of kind words throughout this long process. It was so sweet to hear Noreen say, "Joe is your biggest admirer. If I didn't know better, I would be jealous."

My many thanks go to Dr. Gladys McGarey for writing a profound foreword for this book. As a totally unconventional medical doctor, she challenges us all by posing tough questions about our health care system. Having "the mother of holistic medicine," a pioneer in her own right, be part of my journey is unreal to me. I want to be just like her when I grow up.

A special thanks to Les Brown, Kandee G and Dr. Sonjia for dropping everything to read my book and give me feedback. I still pinch myself when I realize

I have the cell phone numbers of people of their caliber. Again, God has blessed me with great people in my life.

My infinite gratitude to Dr. David Padden, for taking on my case when other doctors sent me away, for his magical surgeon's hands that helped put me back together again, and for never giving up on me. To

Dr. John Coats who, in our one and only meeting, managed to completely change the course of my life.

And to Dr. Scott Denny, the first acupuncture physician who treated me and helped get me back on my feet again after I was bedridden for two years. He was also the first doctor to introduce me to the power of integrative medicine. Without their skills, dedication and willingness to see beyond the obvious, I would not be walking today or writing this book.

Many thanks go to Candice and Yasser Heyaime for selflessly giving their time to help me fulfill my mission in life. There is not enough money in the world to compensate them for their generous contributions of time, talent and support.

Special thanks to Albis Peralta, artist, creative director and graphic designer of Azipra Creatives. His incredible talent is manifested in the design of my logos and marketing materials. His ability to take what is in my head and convert it into a design concept is nothing short of amazing.

Many thanks to all of the practitioners, past and present, at International Holistic Center . They have made it easy for me to write about what excellent health care should look like because they are the epitome of true healers. Also thanks to my dedicated and supportive staff, past and present, for without their willingness to wear many hats, learn lots of new things and cover for me when I was locked away writing, this book would never have happened.

Thanks to Dr. David Webb, Doctor of Oriental Medicine at my center. He has believed and supported my vision from day one. He has helped me develop and perfect my Health Fusion™ protocol, and he is the model of a great doctor and healer.

A special thanks to my friend Yvonne Haase, psychotherapist at my center. She is always ready to tackle with enthusiasm any new project that comes into my head, and she picked up the slack when I was overcommitted so I could write this book. Because of her untiring support and saying "yes" one too many times, we are holding our first Women's International Holistic Conference this year. She has helped make yet another dream of mine come true.

Thanks to Ryan Haase, aka "da-man," another "type A" personality who is a perfectionist. He is the best webmaster on this planet. If I can think it, he can do it; or if not, he is not afraid to go beyond his comfort zone to figure it out. He actually responds to e-mails and understands that when I say "This is urgent!" I mean it. Having him on my team has allowed me to spend more time working on my book.

Miss O'Connor, my special education teacher for grades 2 through 5, taught me that the heart and mind are never handicapped. Because of her, I got to live my own version of my favorite movie "It's a Wonderful Life." Her ability to paint my reality with beautiful colors gave me the confidence to reach for the stars. Even when she visited me in the hospital, put on my leg braces and carried me because I could not walk, she always believed that I would one day be called "doctor" and write books.

Special thanks to my amazing family and friends for all of the prayers and light they send my way. Their love, patience and untiring support are the reasons why I have been able to take on and conquer my life challenges. It would take another entire book just to list all of them and their contributions to my success and this book.

Special thanks to my daughter Elizabeth, who is my inspiration for living. She has contributed to everything I am and hope to be. She has helped me edit and write many papers since she was little, and despite her very busy schedule as a lawyer, she continues to be my editor-in-chief for everything I write. I love her more than life itself.

Special thanks to my sisters, Sandra, Miguelina and Altagracia, for everything they mean to me. They have been there for me through the most difficult times, taking care of and encouraging me without fail. I am so blessed to not only call them my sisters, but also my best friends. My life and this book would not be possible without their unconditional love and support.

Special thanks to my brothers-in-law, Juan, Otto and Sam, for supporting my sisters and me in all of our adventures and craziness. I know that you have sacrificed your time with them so that they could be with me.

Thanks to my stepdaughter, Cory, who has taught me many wonderful lessons in life, including that of forgiving. I love our girl talks and silly times together. I am happy that we have connected in a very special way.

There is no way I can adequately thank my mom, Andrea, the strongest woman I know. She is my role model for what it means to be a great mother, a great philanthropist and a great person. She taught me the true meaning of "attitude is everything." She made me into a survivor, not a victim. Her dedication to her family is unwavering. She has taught me to be fearless.

I am overflowing with gratitude for my husband, soul mate and best friend, John Weaver, and seriously, I do not understand how I am so lucky as to have him in my life. He has stuck by me through many difficult challenges--from surgeries, to being bedridden, to opening up my center, to writing this book.

I remember the days when he would literally get down on his hands and knees to push my feet one step at a time, in what could only be described as an excruciating walk from my bed to the bathroom. He has never complained that it took us almost an hour to go a few yards. He has been my biggest cheerleader and promoter.

I cannot thank him enough for all the times he has brought vitamins and food to me at my computer and said, "This is because I care;" for the times he could not speak because I had a deadline and could not listen; for the many times he has edited and re-edited my papers because I was not happy with them; for the times he has rubbed my legs because they hurt from sitting too long at the computer writing, and for the times he has wiped away my tears when I thought I couldn't go on.

His constant encouragement, untiring support for all that I do, and unconditional love, make me feel so blessed.

Thank you to Mama for selflessly dedicating her life to caring for, loving and encouraging me. She never gave up, even when doctors had lost hope. She went to Heaven insisting that I spoke 23 languages, even after I told her I didn't. She gave me the biggest gift of all, a strong faith in God and the belief that we are all here for a purpose. I know she is smiling in Heaven knowing that I am fulfilling mine.

Thank you to my son-in-law, Brian, for loving my daughter the way she deserves to be loved. For a mother, it is a true blessing to know that your daughter is happy. I love the times we have spent talking about business ventures for hours on end, laughing at YouTube videos, and rapping and dancing. He is the son I never had. I am truly blessed to have him in my life.

Many thanks to Judy and Paul Korchin, Brian's parents, for accepting my daughter as their own. They have with open arms welcomed our family and have selflessly shared their wonderful son. Judy, thank you for introducing me to Noreen. I don't know how I can repay you. I love you both.

I also want to thank all of the angels-in-disguise who have touched my life, whether as a patient, a colleague, a student, a teacher, or a stranger. They have honored me by being part of my journey.

Above all, I want to thank God for the incredible life He has given me. Looking at this long list of acknowledgements, I can only count my blessings, for I have been granted more than my share of opportunities for making a difference, the company of lots of beautiful people, and many wonderful times.

13438285R00084

Made in the USA
Charleston, SC
10 July 2012